Mediterranean Diet Collection

50 Innovative Recipes for your Meals

Sofia Abagnale

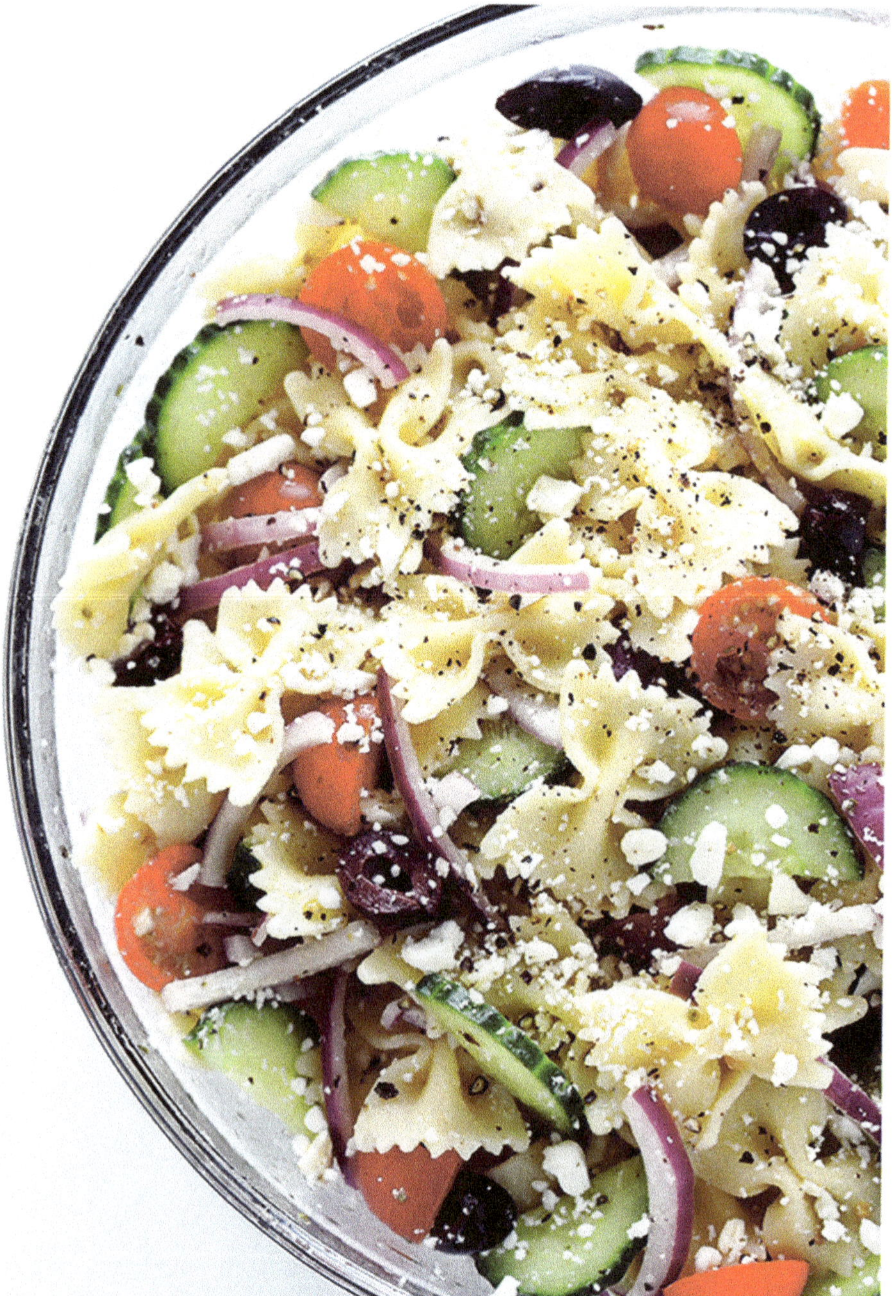

TABLE OF CONTENTS

Tuna fettuccine

Ingredients

- 50g of whole almonds
- 1 x 400g tin of cherry tomatoes
- 30g of pecorino cheese
- 4 baby courgettes with flowers
- 1 small onion
- 2 cloves of garlic
- Extra virgin olive oil
- 4 anchovy fillets in oil
- Olive oil
- 1 lemon
- 300g of dried fettuccine
- 300g of yellowfin tuna

Directions

1. Lightly toast the almonds in a large frying pan on a medium heat.
2. Place into a pestle and mortar.
3. Add onion, garlic, anchovies, olive oil to the pan. Fry for 4 minutes, stirring regularly.
4. Cook the pasta in a pan of boiling salted water according to package Directions.

5. Stir the courgette and tuna into the frying pan.
6. Scrunch in the tomatoes with your hands, and lemon juice, let tick away, stirring regularly.
7. Finely grate the pecorino. Then, Pound the almonds until fine.
8. Once cooked, drag the pasta straight into the frying pan.
9. Toss together, then tear in the courgette flowers and toss in the pecorino with most of the almonds.
10. Taste and adjust the seasoning.
11. Serve and enjoy sprinkled with the remaining almonds.

Jumbo fish fingers

Ingredients

- 30g of Cheddar
- 200g of whole meal bread
- 2kg of salmon
- 2 large free-range eggs
- 100g of plain flour
- Extra virgin olive oil
- 2 teaspoons of sweet smoked paprika

Directions

1. Cut the fish into equal portions
2. Sprinkle the flour across a plate.
3. Then, in a shallow bowl, whisk the eggs together with the paprika and a pinch of sea salt and black pepper.
4. Place the bread into a food processor with the cheese, olive oil, sea salt and black pepper, whisk until breadcrumbs form. Place into a baking tray.
5. Turn each fish portion in the flour to coat.
6. Then, dip in the egg mixture, and later turn it in the breadcrumbs until well coated.

7. Transfer to a baking tray lined with greaseproof paper, layering them up between sheets of paper until all of the fish is coated.
8. Cook immediately or freeze in the tray.
9. To cook, place jumbo fish fingers on the roasting tray, cook in the oven at 400°F for 15 minutes and 20 minutes for fresh and frozen fish respectively.
10. Serve and enjoy when the time is up.

Five-spice salmon tacos

Ingredients

- 2 shallots
- 1 tablespoon of white wine vinegar
- 4 x 125g of salmon fillets, skin on
- 1 fresh red chili
- 1 pinch of sugar
- 3 teaspoons of five spice powder
- 4 corn or flour tortillas
- Olive oil
- ½ a bunch of fresh coriander
- ½ a bunch of fresh mint
- 150g of plain yoghurt
- 1 cucumber

Directions

1. Start by rubbing the salmon flesh with the five spice, a drizzle of olive oil, and a pinch of sea salt and black pepper.
2. Then, heat a frying pan over a medium heat.
3. Place the salmon skin-side down in the pan, let cook for 9 minutes.
4. Remove shortly after flipping.

5. Chop the coriander leaves (reserving a few), and the mint leaves, then combine with the yoghurt.
6. Season to taste.
7. Place cucumber ribbons, shallots, and chili in a bowl, then sprinkle over the vinegar, sugar, and a pinch of salt, and mix with hands to combine.
8. Place a tortilla on each plate and flake over the salmon fillets.
9. Add a dollop of yoghurt, minty cucumber, and reserved coriander leaves.
10. Roll up and enjoy.

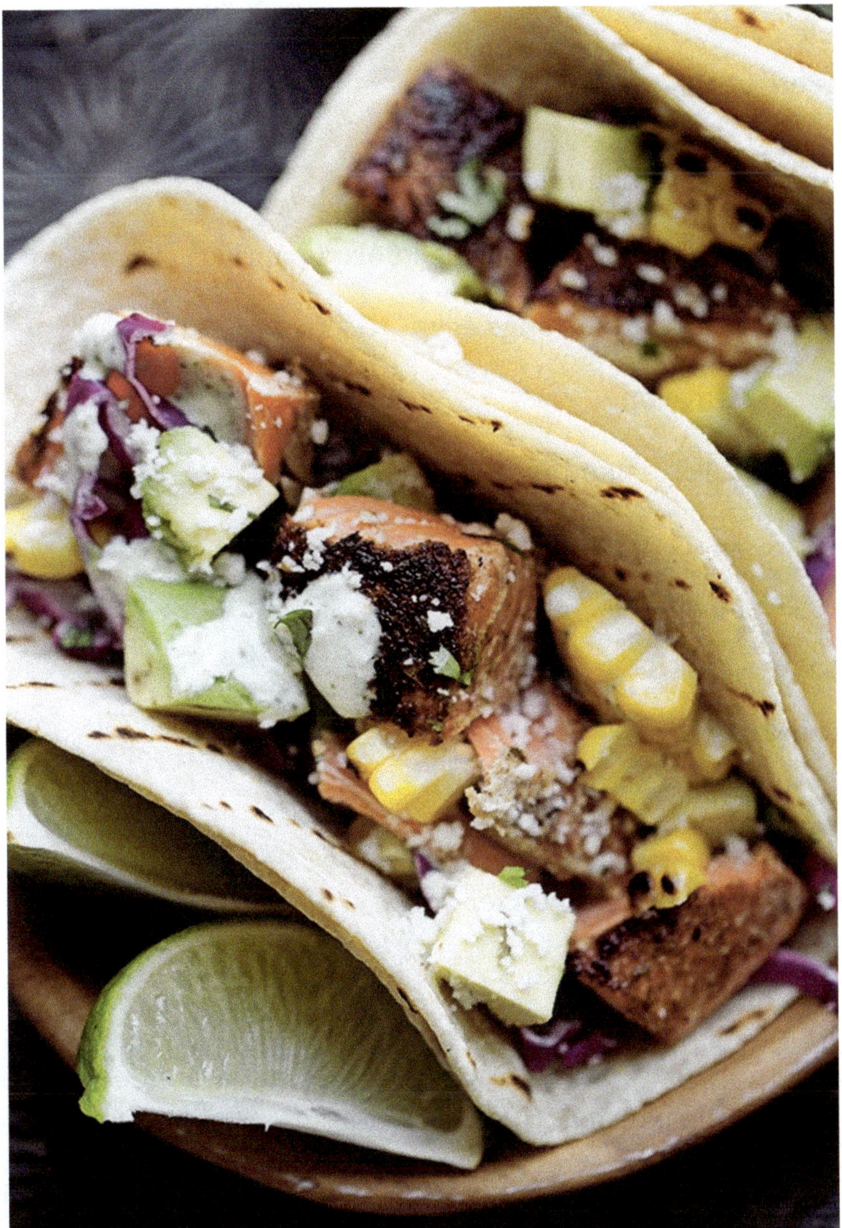

Baked sole goujons

Ingredients

- 50g of plain flour
- 1 tablespoon of sweet smoked paprika
- 2 large free-range eggs
- Olive oil
- 2 large handfuls of breadcrumbs
- 450g of lemon sole fillets

Directions

1. Preheat your oven to 420°F.
2. Cut the fish into finger-width strips.
3. Season the flour and place it on a plate.
4. Crack the eggs into a shallow bowl, and beat lightly.
5. Mix the paprika with the breadcrumbs on another plate.
6. Coat the fish goujons with the seasoned flour, dipping them in the eggs, then coating with the breadcrumbs.

7. Place them on the oiled tray and bake for 15 minutes, until golden.
8. Serve and enjoy with tartare sauce.

Sesame seared salmon

Ingredients

- 2 x 100 g fillets of salmon
- 4 teaspoons of sesame seeds
- 8cm piece of cucumber
- 2 small carrots
- 1 clove of garlic
- 2 sprigs of fresh coriander
- 2 raw baby beets
- 1 punnet of cress
- 150g of brown rice noodles
- 4 teaspoons tahini
- 1 ripe avocado
- Extra virgin olive oil
- 2 limes
- 1 fresh red chili

Directions

1. Cook the noodles according to the packet Directions.
2. Drain and toss in a little squeeze of lime juice.
3. Carefully slice each of the salmon fillets lengthways into three.

4. Scatter the sesame seeds over a board and press one side of the salmon slices into the seeds to form a crust.
5. Place a large dry frying pan over a medium heat, and once hot, add the salmon sesame-side down. Leave for 3 minutes.
6. Pound the garlic with a pinch of sea salt in a pestle and mortar, then muddle in the tahini, the remaining lime juice, and a splash of water to make a wicked dressing.
7. Use a box grater to coarsely grate the cucumber, carrots and beets, keeping them in separate piles and dividing between two plates.
8. Snip and divide up the cress, then divide up the noodles.
9. Add one half of avocado to each plate.
10. Lay the salmon alongside, then finely slice the chili and scatter over with the coriander leaves.
11. Toss everything together at the table.
12. Serve and enjoy.

Sicilian fish soup

Ingredients

- ½ lemon
- 1 red onion
- 2 sticks celery
- 1 large handful fresh flat-leaf parsley, chopped
- ½ small bulb fennel
- 2 cloves garlic
- ½ butternut squash, peeled and grated
- 1 red chili, deseeded
- 200g of salmon fillet
- 12 raw peeled prawns or langoustine tails
- 300g of halibut fillet
- 2 tablespoons of olive oil
- 1 glass of dry white wine
- 800g of chopped plum tomatoes
- 500ml of organic fish stock

Directions

1. Finely chop the onion, celery, fennel, garlic and chili.
2. Then, heat the oil in a large pan.
3. Add the onion together with the celery, fennel, garlic, and chili and sweat gently until soft.

4. Add the wine, tomatoes or passata, squash, and stock and bring to the boil.
5. Cover and simmer gently for 30 minutes.
6. Season and gently break up the tomatoes.
7. Roughly chop the salmon and halibut and add to the pan.
8. Add the prawns or langoustine tails, cover and simmer for 10 minutes.
9. Taste the soup and season and adjust.
10. Serve and enjoy drizzled with olive oil and sprinkled with the chopped parsley.

Carbonara of smoked mackerel

Ingredient

- 2 sprigs of fresh rosemary
- 320g of dried penne
- 2 large eggs
- 1 lemon
- 40g of Parmesan cheese
- 1 onion
- 1 large courgette
- 100ml of semi-skimmed milk
- 130g of smoked boneless mackerel fillets
- Olive oil

Directions

1. Cook the penne in a pan of boiling salted water as instructed on the package.
2. Place the onions together with the courgettes into a large frying pan on a medium heat with olive oil.
3. Season with a pinch of sea salt and black pepper, stirring occasionally.
4. Add the rosemary with the mackerel after 5 minutes, let cook for a further 5 minutes, tossing occasionally.

5. Then, whisk the eggs and milk together, then grate in the Parmesan.
6. Drain the pasta once ready, reserving some water for later, toss into a mackerel pan.
7. Remove the pan briefly, stir in splash of the reserved water to cool it down.
8. Quickly pour in the egg mixture, stir until thickened, and evenly coated.
9. Serve and enjoy with an extra grating of Parmesan.

Mighty mackerel

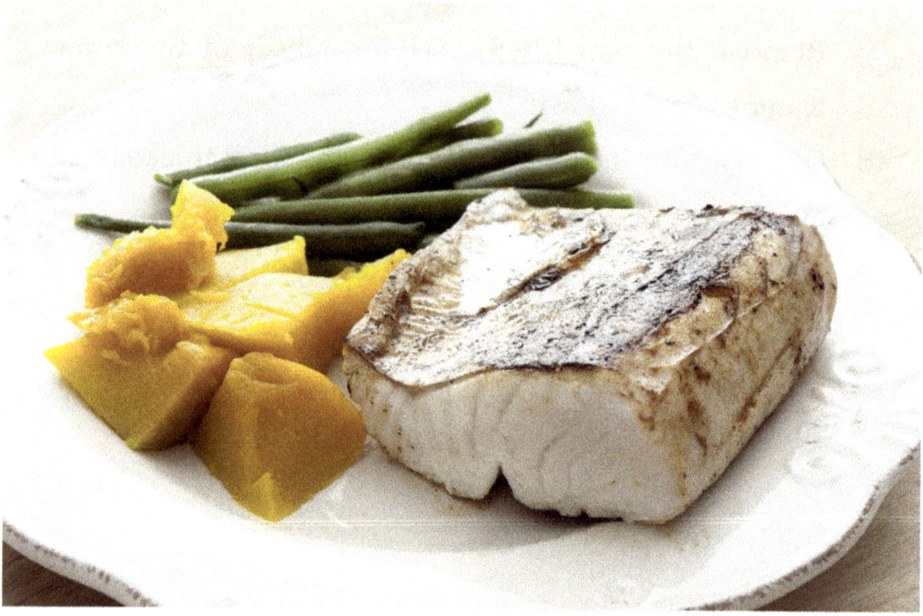

Ingredients

- 2 heaped teaspoons of jarred grated horseradish
- 1 heaped teaspoon of ground coriander
- 1 mug of quinoa
- 2 sprigs of fresh rosemary
- ½ a lemon
- A few sprigs of fresh basil
- 800g of ripe mixed-color tomatoes
- 1 fresh red chili
- 2 tablespoons of extra virgin olive oil

- 2 heaped tablespoons of natural yoghurt
- 2 cloves of garlic
- 1 tablespoon of balsamic vinegar
- 4 x 200g of whole mackerel
- Olive oil

Directions

1. Place the quinoa, pinch of sea salt, lemon half, and 2 mugs of boiling water into the medium pan, cover, stir frequently.
2. Then, score the mackerel on both sides down to the bone on a greaseproof paper.
3. Rub all over with salt, black pepper and the ground coriander.
4. Place into the large frying pan with bit of olive oil.
5. Arrange tomatoes on a large board and sprinkle over with the chili.
6. Strip the rosemary leaves over the fish, then add the whole garlic cloves.
7. Turn the fish when golden.
8. Drain the quinoa when ready, squeeze the lemon juice over it.
9. Spoon the quinoa into the center of the tomatoes.
10. Drizzle with 2 tablespoons of extra virgin olive oil, balsamic, and a pinch of salt and pepper.

11. Then, lay the crispy fish on top.
12. Mix the yoghurt with the horseradish
13. Serve and enjoy.

Mackerel plaki

Ingredients

- 4 sprigs of fresh flat-leaf parsley
- 8 small whole mackerel
- 3 fresh bay leaves
- 3 teaspoons of extra virgin olive oil
- 2 carrots
- 150ml of dry white wine
- 2 onions
- 4 ripe tomatoes
- 3 cloves of garlic
- 1 lemon

Directions

1. Preheat the oven to 350°F.
2. Peel and thinly slice the carrots, then peel and slice the onions.
3. Roughly chop the tomatoes and finely chop the cloves of garlic.
4. Place the fish together with the onion, tomato, carrot, garlic, and bay leaves in a baking dish.
5. Season with sea salt and black pepper, then drizzle over the oil.

6. Sprinkle the chopped parsley over the fish.
7. Squeeze in the lemon juice, then, add the wine and a little water.
8. Let bake for 30 minutes or until the sauce has thickened.
9. Serve and enjoy with an extra squeeze of lemon.

Pan-cooked asparagus mixed with fish

Ingredients

- 1 small handful of thyme tips
- Olive oil
- Extra virgin olive oil
- 2 small red mullet
- 1 lemon
- 1 royal bream fillet
- 2 small squid
- 4 freshly shelled scallops
- 1 small handful of fennel tops
- 10 medium asparagus spears
- 1 fresh red chili

Directions

1. Place a large frying pan to heat with olive oil.
2. Score the skin of the fish fillets and season.
3. Place the fillets into the pan, skin side down, with the squid tentacles.
4. Add the scallops.

5. Then, run your knife down one side of each squid to open them out.
6. Slightly score the inside in a crisscross fashion.
7. Lay in the pan, scored side down.
8. Add the asparagus, gently shake the pan.
9. Cook briefly, then turn everything over and cook the other side.
10. Sprinkle over the thyme tips.
11. When the fish and scallops turn golden on the edges, remove the pan.
12. Place the squid on a chopping board, slice into pieces, then return to the pan.
13. Lay the fish fillets on each plate.
14. Toss the asparagus, scallops, and squid with half the chili and a good drizzle of extra virgin olive oil.
15. Taste and season accordingly.
16. Divide on top of the plated fish.
17. Sprinkle with the rest of the chopped chili and the fennel tops.
18. Serve and enjoy with extra virgin olive oil.

Peruvian seafood stew with cilantro broth

Ingredients

- 1 green bell pepper
- 6 cloves garlic
- • 1 tablespoon of coriander
- 2 teaspoons of cumin
- 2 lbs. seafood
- 4 cups of chicken broth
- 2 tablespoons olive oil
- 3 cups of water
- 4 cups of small diced potatoes
- 1 yellow or white onion
- Juice of 3 limes
- 2 cup of diced carrots
- ½ teaspoon of cracked pepper
- 2 whole bunches of cilantro
- 1 fresh green ancho chili
- 1 teaspoon of kosher salt

Directions

1. Heat oil over medium high heat.

2. Add onion, let sauté for 3 minutes, stirring often.
3. Add ancho chili with bell pepper.
4. Add garlic with spices, cook briefly until fragrant.
5. Transfer to a blender , set aside.
6. In the same pot, add 4 cups of chicken broth and water boil.
7. Add the small diced potatoes and carrots, simmer over medium heat for 10 minutes.
8. Add two whole bunches of cilantro to the blender , with water, blend until smooth. Keep for later.
9. Add all the seafood simmer for 3 minutes.
10. Stir in blended cilantro mixture from the blender .
11. Season and adjust accordingly.
12. Serve and enjoy.

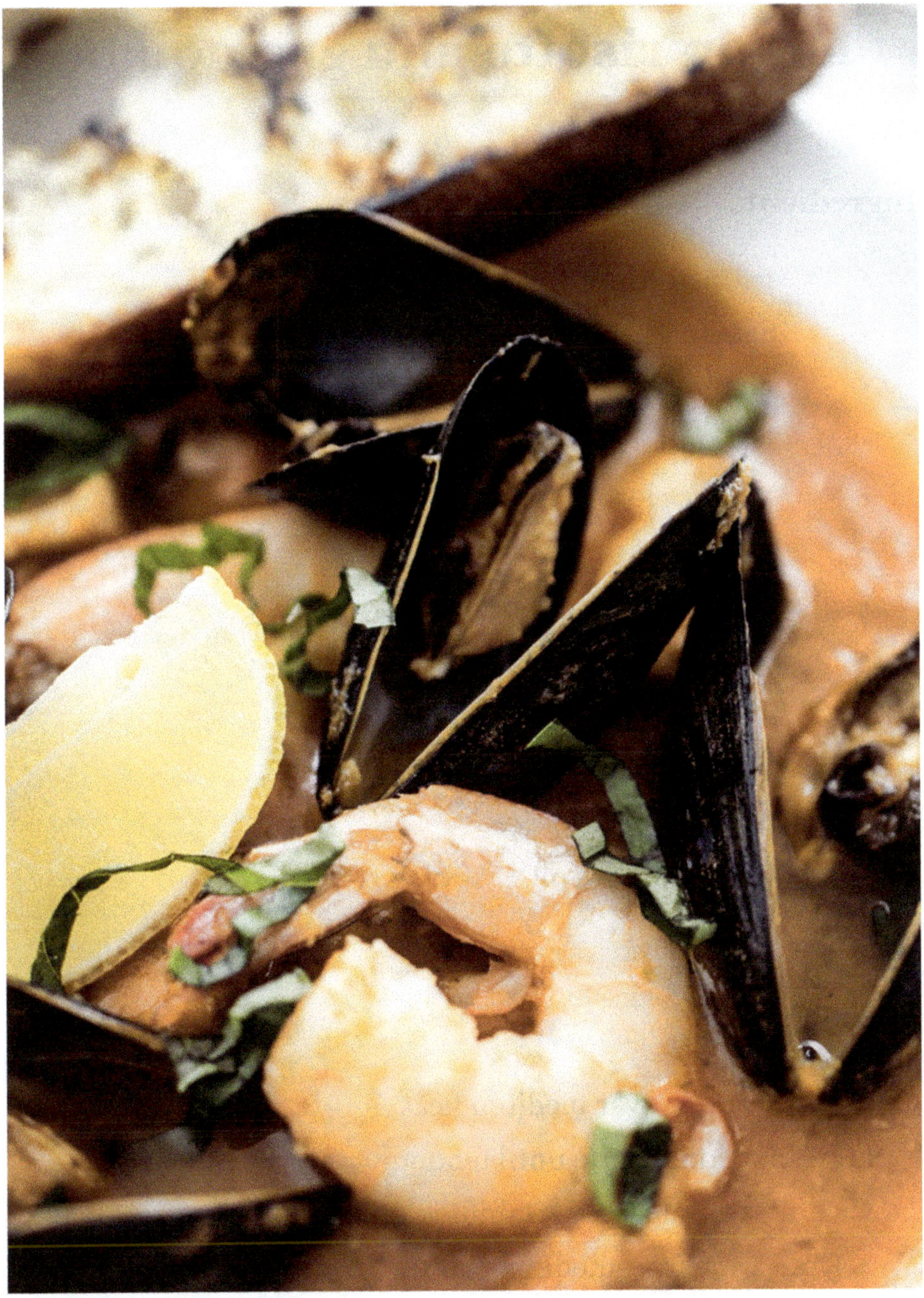

Seared black cod with Meyer lemon risotto and gremolata

Ingredients

- 1 cup of white onion, finely diced
- Salt and pepper
- 1 cup white wine
- 1-pound filet of Black Cod
- 1 garlic clove- finely minced
- 5 cups hot water or stock
- 2 tablespoons of butter or oil
- ¼ teaspoon of white pepper
- 3 Meyer lemons, juice and zest
- ½ cup of chopped Italian parsley
- 2 cups of aborio rice
- ½ cup of olive oil

Directions

1. Melt butter over medium heat.
2. Add onions, sauté until tender.
3. Add rice, sauté for 5 minutes, stirring often.
4. Add wine over medium-low and stir to absorb.

5. Add ½ cup of hot water and stir to absorb for 20 minutes over low heat.
6. Season with salt , white pepper , and zest.
7. Combine parsley, lemon juice, olive oil, garlic and salt.
8. Heat olive oil over medium high heat.
9. Pat dry fish and season.
10. Place skin side down in the skillet and sear.
11. Continue searing over low heat for 5 minutes, until skin is crisp.
12. Serve and enjoy with roasted asparagus.

Grilled fish tacos with cilantro lime cabbage slaw

Ingredients

- ½ cup chopped cilantro
- ½ of a jalapeño
- 1 ½ teaspoon of chili powder
- ¼ cup fresh lime juice
- 1 teaspoon of cumin
- 2 tablespoon of olive oil
- 1 teaspoon of coriander
- 1 teaspoon of granulated garlic
- ½ teaspoon of sugar
- 2 lbs. of grill able white fish
- ¼ teaspoon of chipotle powder
- 3/4 teaspoon of kosher salt
- 1 pound of thinly sliced or shredded cabbage
- ¼ cup of thinly sliced red onion

Directions

1. Preheat your grill ready to medium heat.
2. Place the shredded cabbage in a medium bowl. Toss with the salt .

3. Add onions together with cilantro, lime juice, jalapeño, olive oil and toss well.
4. Grill each side briefly, letting grill marks develop, flip to grill the other side.
5. Grill the tortillas, brush with olive oi
6. Serve and enjoy.

Quick and easy salmon cakes

Ingredients

- Salt and pepper
- 1 egg
- 2 tablespoons sour cream
- 3 tablespoon of mayo
- 1 teaspoon of lemon juice
- 2 tablespoons fresh dill
- Squeeze of lemon
- ½ teaspoon of garlic powder
- 1 can of salmon
- ⅓ cup of toasted bread crumbs
- 2 scallions, sliced
- Olive oil for searing

Directions

1. Mix all ingredients together in a medium bowl. Let settle for 10 minutes.
2. Divide mixture into 2 larger cakes pressing together with your hands.
3. Heat oil in a skillet over medium heat.
4. Sear the salmon cakes for 5 minutes on each side until golden.

5. Serve with the quick creamy sauce.
6. Enjoy.

Balinese fish and potato curry

Ingredients

- Sambal oelek
- 12 ounces of while fish
- 1 tablespoon of fresh turmeric
- 2 x 5 inch stocks lemongrass
- 1 cup of peas
- 3 garlic cloves
- 1 tablespoon of fish sauce
- 1 jalapeno
- 5 kefir lime leaves
- 2 tablespoons of coconut oil
- 2 cups of water
- 10 ounces of baby potatoes
- 2 tablespoons of thinly sliced ginger
- 1 can of coconut milk
- ½ teaspoon of salt
- 1 shallot rough chopped
- 1 lime- juice

Directions

1. Cook rice as instructed on the package.

2. Place the thinly sliced ginger together with the lemongrass, shallot, and turmeric in the food processor .
3. Add the jalapeño, garlic, and lime leaves. Pulse to foam.
4. Heat coconut oil over medium high heat.
5. Add the paste and stir constantly for 4 minutes.
6. Add and boil 2 cups of water.
7. Add potatoes, cover let simmer for 15 minutes.
8. Add coconut milk with salt , fish sauce and lime juice
9. Taste, and adjust accordingly.
10. Place the fish into the coconut sauce and simmer for 5 minutes.
11. Place in the spring peas cook briefly.
12. Serve and enjoy with lime wedges.

Pasty's garlic and chili prawns

Ingredients

- ½ teaspoon of smoked paprika
- 1 lemon
- 3 cloves of garlic
- 1 fresh red chili
- 8 large raw shell-on king prawns
- Sprigs of fresh flat-leaf parsley
- 50ml of olive oil

Directions

1. Drizzle oil into a shallow heatproof terracotta dish over a medium-high heat.
2. Add garlic with chili and fry briefly.
3. Stir in the paprika.
4. Add the prawns and parsley, fry for 2 minutes on each side.

5. Squeeze half the lemon juice into the dish.
6. Remove and sprinkle over the remaining parsley and a pinch of sea salt.
7. Serve and enjoy with lemon wedges.

Paella

Ingredients

- 500g of paella rice
- 6 free-range chicken thighs
- 1 heaped teaspoon of smoked paprika
- 500g of mussel
- olive oil
- 100g of quality chorizo
- 10 large raw shell-on king prawns
- 1 onion
- 1 lemon
- 4 cloves of garlic
- Plain flour
- ½ a bunch of fresh flat-leaf parsley
- 6 rashers of higher-welfare pancetta
- 2 liters of organic chicken stock
- 2 handfuls of fresh or frozen peas
- 2 large pinches of saffron
- 2 small squid

Directions

1. Preheat the oven to 375°F.

2. Heat a splash of oil over medium heat, fry the chicken until golden brown.
3. Bake for 20 minutes.
4. Return the pan to heat, add chorizo and pancetta, fry until browned.
5. Add the onion together with the garlic and parsley stalks, cook until soft.
6. Heat and infuse the chicken stock with the saffron.
7. Add the smoked paprika, rice and infused stock to the pan, let cook for around 20 minutes on low heat.
8. Add the remaining stock, peas, prawns, and the mussels, let cook for 10 minutes.
9. Add the cooked chicken, sprinkle over the chopped parsley.
10. Serve and enjoy with wedges.

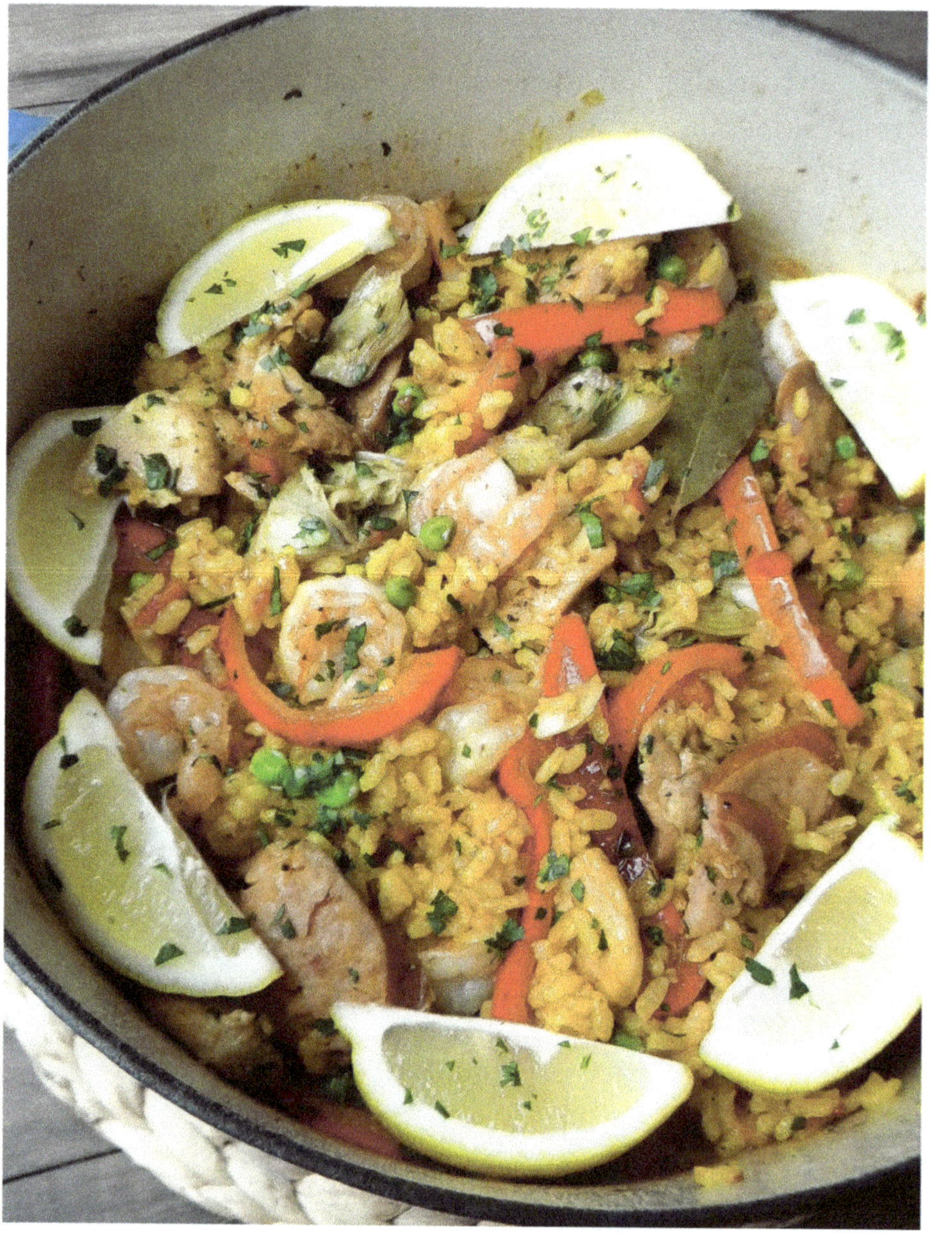

Retro crab cocktail

Ingredients

- 1 tablespoon of tomato ketchup
- ¼ of a cucumber
- Cayenne pepper
- 1 lemon
- 1 ripe avocado
- 6 radishes
- 300g of cooked white crab meat
- 1 punnet of cress
- 1 punnet of micro herbs
- ½ of an iceberg lettuce
- 3 tablespoons of mayonnaise
- 1 teaspoon of Worcestershire sauce

Directions

1. Mix the mayo, ketchup, and Worcestershire sauce in a bowl.
2. Add lemon juice with brandy.
3. Season with sea salt and black pepper.
4. Mix the crabmeat with the mayo
5. Divide the crab between the plates and drizzle over a little Marie Rose sauce.

6. Serve and enjoy.

Seared tuna steak

Ingredients

- 1 handful of fresh coriander
- 1 small dried red chili
- Tuna steaks
- 1 tablespoon of coriander seeds
- 1 lemon
- ½ clove of garlic
- 1 handful of fresh basil
- Olive oil

Directions

1. Combine the garlic, herb leaves, olive oil, and lemon juice, mix in a mortar.
2. Season with salt and pepper.
3. Lay out the tuna steaks on a tray, season both sides, rub with the herb mixture.
4. Place in the tuna, toasts and fry for 60 seconds on each side.
5. Serve and enjoy with potatoes.

Honeymoon spaghetti

Ingredients

- 1 large free-range egg
- 5 cloves of garlic
- 1 fresh red chili
- 1 fresh red chili
- 450g of mussels
- 1.5kg of crab
- 100g of squid
- 2 x 400g tins of plum tomatoes
- 30g of unsalted butter
- 200g of raw shell-off tiger prawns
- 450g of dried spaghetti
- 1 bunch of flat-leaf parsley
- 1 bunch of marjoram
- 3 cloves of garlic

Directions

1. Preheat the oven to 350°F.
2. Boil crab for 15 minutes, let cool.
3. Remove the meat, flake into small pieces.
4. Combine pounded shells with chopped garlic.
5. Drizzle with olive oil over a medium heat and fry.

6. Add the broken tomatoes with water, simmer for 1 hour.
7. Sieve, season with sea salt and black pepper.
8. Cook the spaghetti as instructed on the package. Drain.
9. Melt the butter with olive oil. Add garlic and chili to the pan, fry. S
10. Raise the heat, then mussel prawns let cook for 2 minutes.
11. Remove from the heat, discard unopened mussels.
12. Add tomato sauce, pasta parsley, marjoram leaves, and crab, mix.
13. Place the seafood mixture in the center of a baking tray, beat the egg.
14. Use it to brush the edges, seal and cook for 10 minutes.
15. Serve and enjoy.

Seafood risotto

Ingredients

- ½ a bunch of fresh rosemary
- Olive oil
- 6 raw langoustines
- 1.6 liters quality fish stock
- 300g of mussels, scrubbed
- Extra virgin olive oil
- 400g of risotto rice
- 500g of clams, scrubbed
- 2 cloves of garlic
- 4 medium squid
- 300g of cooked white crab meat
- 1 knob of butter
- 1 pinch of saffron
- 400g of mixed cherry tomatoes
- 1 large onion
- 1 heart of celery
- 1 bulb of fennel
- ½ a glass of white wine
- 30g of Parmesan cheese

Directions

1. Preheat the oven to 325°F.
2. Tip tomatoes into a medium roasting tray.
3. Combine garlic, rosemary leaves, tomatoes, olive oil and toss to coat and space them out in a single layer.
4. Let roast for 40 minutes
5. Put the saffron in a small bowl, cover with 50ml of freshly boiled water, infuse.
6. Place onion, celery, fennel in a pan with oil over a medium heat, let cook for 15 minutes, stir in the rice, toast for 2 minutes.
7. Pour in the wine, and stir until absorbed.
8. Add a ladleful of stock, let it be fully absorbed.
9. Add the saffron and its soaking liquid, stir in the mussels with clams.
10. Beat in the butter, Parmesan, season.
11. Dot over the roasted tomatoes and herbs.
12. Serve and enjoy.

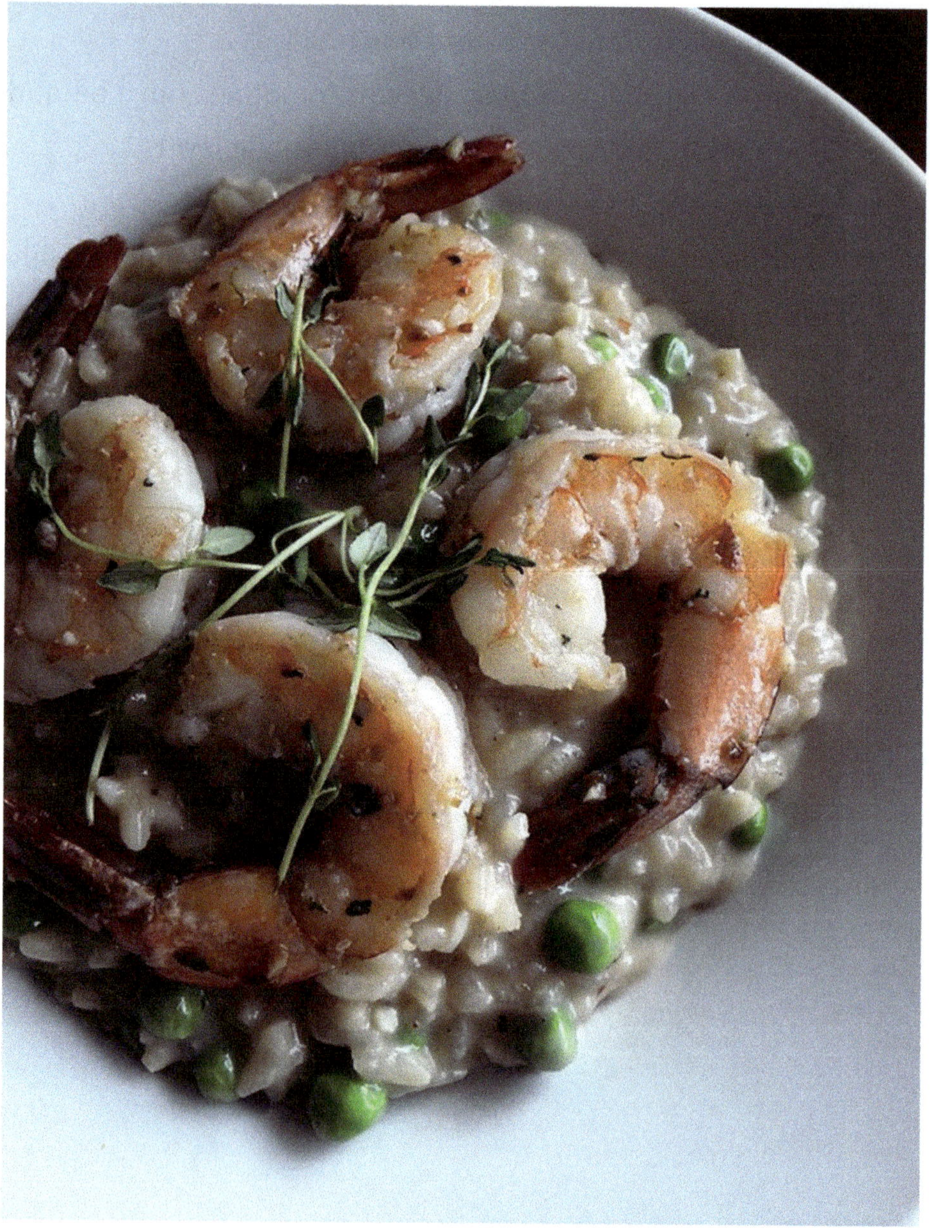

Grilled squid salad

Ingredients

- ½ a bunch of fresh mint
- 2 tablespoons of baby capers in brine
- 500g of large ripe tomatoes
- 2 lemons
- Extra virgin olive oil
- 4 large squid
- 1 clove of garlic
- 30g of shelled unsalted pistachios
- 1 fresh red chili
- 4 anchovy fillets in oil

Directions

1. Combine garlic, chili, anchovies, pistachios, capers, and mint leaves in a mixing bowl. Mix well.
2. Add the tubes, from largest to smallest. Cook each piece for about 1 minute per side.
3. As each piece is done, use tongs to dunk it straight into the salsa, turning and coating it in flavor.
4. Slice the tomatoes and lay over a serving platter.
5. Slice the squid tubes, pull the tentacles apart, then arrange on top of the tomatoes.

6. Serve and enjoy.

Stuffed braised squid

Ingredients

- 25g of baby capers in brine
- 4 medium squid
- 300g of dried spaghetti
- 1 x 680g jar of passata
- 100g of coarse stale breadcrumbs
- 2 sprigs of fresh basil
- Olive oil
- 15g of pecorino
- 1 clove of garlic
- ½ a bunch of fresh flat-leaf parsley
- 1 red onion
- 1 large free-range egg
- 10 ripe cherry tomatoes

Directions

1. Place half the capers in a bowl with the breadcrumbs, garlic, pecorino, egg, olive oil and water, mix.
2. Combine onions, tomatoes, add to pan with passata and let Simmer on a low heat.
3. Fill squid tubes with breadcrumb mixture seal with toothpick.

4. Stir the remaining capers into the sauce, with stuffed squid and tentacles.
5. Simmer on a low heat for 25 minutes, or until tender.
6. cook the pasta according to the packet Directions.
7. Transfer the squid to board. Arrange.
8. Serve and enjoy.

Prawn and tuna linguine

Ingredients

- 150g of dried linguine
- 4 large raw shell-on prawns
- Olive oil
- 2 small onions
- 1 cinnamon stick
- ½ a bunch of fresh flat-leaf parsley
- 1 good pinch of saffron
- 200g of yellowfin tuna
- 4 tablespoons white wine vinegar
- 2 anchovy fillets in oil
- 50g of shelled unsalted pistachios
- Pecorino or Parmesan cheese rind

Directions

1. Over medium heat, place onions, prawn heads, olive oil, and cinnamon in a pan.
2. Add anchovies once sizzling. Drain, toss.
3. Cook for 20 minutes when covered as you stir occasionally.
4. Cook the pasta according to the packet Directions.

5. Gently squash each prawn head so all the tasty juices spill out into the pan.
6. Stir in half the parsley, prawns, tuna, and saffron vinegar mixture.
7. Drag the pasta straight into the pan, letting a little starchy cooking water go with it.
8. Toss for 2 minutes.
9. Season accordingly.
10. Serve and enjoy.

Smoked salmon pate

Ingredients

- 2 lemons
- 150g of cooked peeled prawns
- 150g of quality smoked salmon
- 1 celery heart
- ½ a bunch of fresh dill
- 150g of white crabmeat
- 1 fresh red chili
- 1 loaf of sourdough bread
- 280g of cream cheese
- 25g of salmon caviar
- 1 lemon
- Extra virgin olive oil
- Cayenne pepper
- 1 small red onion

Directions

1. Place the prawns with smoked fish in a bowl with the crabmeat, grated zest, cream cheese, caviar, and black pepper mix well.
2. Spoon into a dish and smooth out evenly.
3. Place into the fridge until needed.

4. Combine red onion, chili, celery, leaves, dill, and lemon wedges and refrigerate overnight.
5. Slice and toast the bread.
6. Cut a crisscross pattern into the top of the pâté.
7. Drizzle with a little oil and sprinkle with a pinch of cayenne.
8. Serve and enjoy.

Chipotle fried fish and clementine bites

Ingredients

- 75g of plain yoghurt
- 400g of white fish fillets
- 2 limes
- 1 teaspoon dried chipotle flakes
- 2 clementine
- 1 liter of vegetable oil
- ½ of a clementine
- 1 teaspoon ground coriander
- ½ a bunch of fresh coriander
- 150g of corn flour
- 1 small clove of garlic
- 150ml of milk

Directions

1. Season the chopped fish with sea salt and black pepper, squeeze over the juice of 1 lime. keep aside for 10 minutes.
2. Stir coriander leaves through the yoghurt in a small bowl.
3. Add garlic and zest of the clementine.

4. In a shallow dish combine ground coriander, corn flour and a pinch of salt, mix well.
5. Pour the milk into a separate bowl.
6. Heat olive oil
7. Pat the fish and clementine slices coat with corn flour, dip briefly in the milk.
8. Coat again and shake off any excess.
9. Deep fry the fish and clementine for 3 minutes.
10. Drain any excess oil, scatter with salt, chipotle and the reserved coriander.
11. Serve and enjoy immediately.

Crispy Mediterranean Sea base

Ingredients

- 1 lime
- 2 x 300g of whole sea bass
- 4 spring onions
- 2 tablespoons of red curry paste
- ½ a bunch of fresh coriander

Directions

1. Place a large non-stick frying pan on a medium temperature.
2. Place onions in ice cold water to crisp.
3. Pack the coriander stalks into the cavities
4. Season with sea salt and black pepper, place in the hot pan with olive oil.
5. Let cook for 4 minutes per side.
6. Drain and shake off the spring onions and coriander.

7. Sit the sea bass on top, spooning over any spicy oil from the pan.
8. Serve and enjoy.

Smoked salmon, prawns and Miami cocktail sauce

Ingredients

- 2 tablespoons of chili sauce
- 2cm of piece of ginger
- Sprigs of fresh coriander
- 4 tablespoons of tomato ketchup
- 3 baby gem lettuces
- 300g of smoked salmon
- 24 large cooked peeled prawns
- 1 lime
- 1 teaspoon of English mustard
- ½ a large clove of garlic
- Extra virgin olive oil
- 1 spring onion
- 4 tablespoons of free-range mayonnaise

Directions

1. Combine garlic, spring onion, coriander leaves, mayonnaise, tomato ketchup, chili, ginger, and mustard. Mix.
2. Place in the fridge for 1 hour.

3. Drape the lettuce over the smoked salmon, organize the prawns on top.
4. Dress the lettuce and seafood with the cocktail sauce.
5. Cut the lime into wedges and squeeze a little juice over each plate.
6. Serve and enjoy with black pepper.

Roasted scallops with pancetta and hazelnuts

Ingredients

- 150g of hazelnuts
- 4 scallops in the half shell
- 1 small onion
- 1 sprig of fresh tarragon
- 80g of pancetta
- 2 cloves of garlic
- Olive oil

Directions

1. Preheat the oven to 350°F.
2. Place a frying pan over a medium heat and drizzle with a little oil.
3. Add the pancetta, garlic, and onion let fry until golden.
4. Toast and roughly chop the hazelnuts with tarragon, place on one side.
5. Divide the pancetta mixture between the scallops, pouring any juices from the pan over the top.
6. Bake in the preheated oven 7 minutes, or until the flesh is no longer translucent.

7. Sprinkle the chopped hazelnuts over the scallops
8. Serve and enjoy with tarragon leaves.

Pesto mussel and toast

Ingredients

- 160g of fresh or frozen peas
- 70g of pesto
- 500g of mussels, scrubbed, debarred
- 2 thick slices of whole meal bread
- 2 sprigs of fresh basil
- 200g of baby courgettes
- 200g of ripe mixed-color cherry tomatoes
- 50ml of white wine

Directions

1. Heat a large pan on a medium-high heat.
2. Toast the bread as the pan heats up.
3. Remove the toast and spread one quarter of the pesto on each slice of courgrette and tomatoes.
4. Raise the heat, place in the mussels.
5. Stir in the remaining pesto, courgettes, tomatoes, and peas.
6. Add the wine and steam for 4 minutes, shaking the pan occasionally.
7. Serve and enjoy.

Roasted razor clams

Ingredients

- 2 fresh red chilies
- 2 lemons
- Olive oil
- 3 cloves of garlic
- 3 sprigs of fresh rosemary
- 1kg of razor clams

Directions

1. Preheat the oven to oven to high.
2. Spread the clams in a roasting tray.
3. Spread the sliced chilies, garlic, rosemary, and drizzle with olive oil.
4. Let roast for 6 minutes.
5. Remove and add lemon juice.
6. Drizzle with extra virgin olive oil and serve with crusty bread.
7. Enjoy.

Fried clams with rice noodles

Ingredients

- 3 kaffir lime leaves
- 1 kg clams
- 2 teaspoons of fish sauce
- 220g of rice noodles
- 5cm piece of galangal
- 2 limes
- 1 shallot
- 6 red chilies
- 1 tablespoon of rice vinegar
- ½ a bunch of fresh coriander
- Olive oil
- 2 tablespoons red chili paste

Directions

1. Cook the noodles as per package Directions. Drain and set aside.
2. Combine the clams and noodles in a saucepan over a medium heat.
3. Add fry the chili paste briefly, add the galangal, chilies, shallots, and coriander until the shallots soften.

4. Add the clams and lime leaves, fry briefly then add the vinegar with bit of water.
5. Let cook over a high heat for 2 to 3 minutes covered until all the clams have opened.
6. Remove and stir in the noodles, clams, fish sauce, and the juice from 1 lime.
7. Let sit for a couple of minutes.
8. Serve and enjoy with lime wedges.

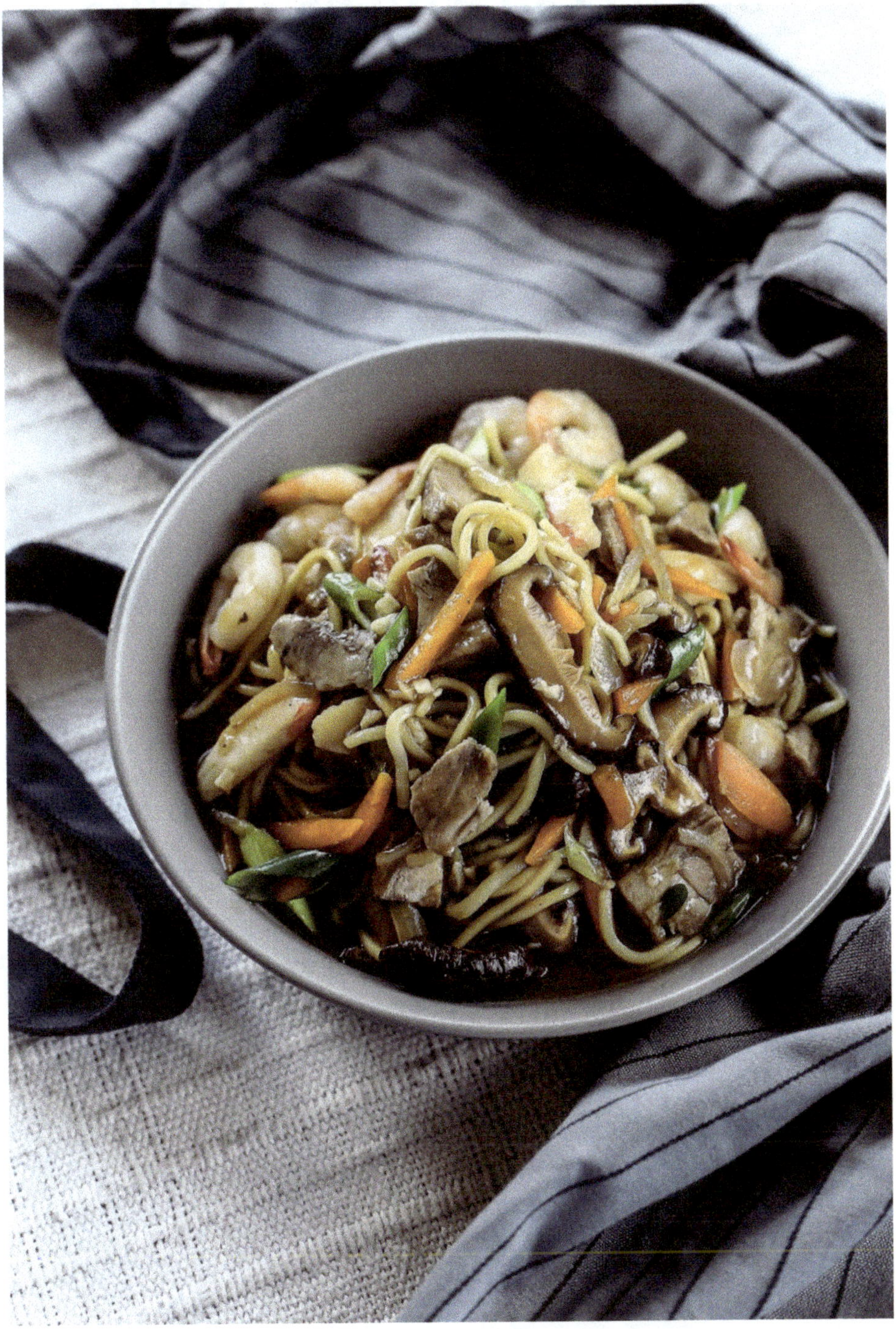

Potted crab with asparagus

Ingredients

- 1 good pinch of ground mace
- 1 fresh red chili
- 225g of unsalted butter
- Sprigs of fresh dill
- 300g of fresh crabmeat
- 1 good pinch of ground cayenne
- 1 whole nutmeg
- 1 Sicilian lemon

Directions

1. In a bowl, mix the crab together with the mace, cayenne and nutmeg, lemon zest and juice, chili, and a pinch of sea salt, mix in 125g of the butter.
2. Spoon into a small serving bowl, smoothing the surface.
3. Scatter with the dill over the top.
4. Melt the remaining butter, spoon the clarified butter over the crab.
5. Cover and refrigerate for 10 hours until set.
6. Serve and enjoy with hot sourdough toasts.

Oyster Rockefeller

Ingredients

- Drops of Tabasco
- 1 small handful of stale breadcrumbs
- 500g of rock salt
- 1 tablespoon of butter
- 3 spring onions
- 6 oysters in deep shells
- 1 stick of celery
- Sprigs of fresh tarragon

Directions

1. Place the shells with oyster on a bed of rock salt in baking tray.
2. Place spring onions and celery in a food processor with tarragon leaves, and the remaining ingredients.
3. Blend to a paste.
4. Season, then spoon a little on top of each oyster.
5. Cook under a hot grill for 10 minutes.
6. Serve and enjoy.

Sticky sesame prawns

The sticky sesame prawns feature great flavors from ginger, garlic, chili, miso, and spring onions perfect for a Mediterranean Sea diet.

Ingredients

- 3 cloves of garlic
- 200ml of fresh cloudy apple juice
- 1 bunch of fresh coriander
- 100g of snow peas
- 2 tablespoons of runny honey
- 200g of tender stem broccoli
- 300g of fine rice noodles
- 3 limes
- 2 carrots
- 1 tablespoon of sweet miso
- 2 tablespoons of sesame seeds
- Vegetable oil
- 16 large raw shell-on green banana king prawns
- 2 spring onions
- ½ of a cucumber
- 1 fresh red chili
- 5cm piece of ginger

- 2 spring onions
- 2 tablespoons of hot chili sauce

Directions

1. Place the ginger, garlic, apple juice, miso, honey, and chili sauce and onions in a medium pan. Let boil.
2. Lower the heat, let simmer for 5 minutes.
3. Cook the rice noodles according to the packet Directions.
4. Add the broccoli to blanch with the rice noodles. Drain and toss in sauce and the juice of 2 limes.
5. Toast the sesame seeds in a small pan over a medium heat for 3 minutes.
6. Heat a splash of olive oil, add the whole prawns and stir-fry for 3 minutes.
7. Pour in the remaining sauce, let cook for a further 2 minutes.
8. Serve and enjoy with lime wedges.

Spring ahi with new potatoes, dill sauce, yogurt, and chive blossoms

Ingredients

- 8 ounces of ahi
- 1 teaspoon of fennel seeds
- ½ cup of water
- 2 tablespoons of coconut
- ½ teaspoon of kosher salt
- ¼ cup of light olive oil
- 2 ounces of baby spinach
- 1 ounce of dill
- 8 ounces of baby potatoes
- 1 scallion, chopped
- ¼ teaspoon of kosher salt
- 2 teaspoons of lemon juice
- ½ teaspoon of black pepper
- 1 tablespoon of coriander seeds

Directions

1. Place potatoes in a small pot , boil over high heat.

2. Simmer until fork tender for 25 minutes.
3. Blend water, olive oil and spinach.
4. Add dill with scallion, salt and pepper and blend until smooth.
5. Taste, and adjust.
6. Place seeds, salt and pepper on a small plate and mix well.
7. Coat ahi with the seed mixture.
8. Heat oil over medium high heat.
9. Fry for 2 minutes, until golden brown crust.
10. Turn over, and cook for 1 minute.
11. Serve and enjoy.

Outlaw seafood burger

Ingredients

- 50g of fresh English wasabi
- Pickled onions
- 2 cloves of garlic
- 300ml of sunflower oil
- 1 fresh green chili
- olive oil
- 200g of cod fillet, skinned and pin-boned
- 100g of fresh white and brown crabmeat
- 1 small handful of rocket
- 100g of raw king prawns
- 2 baby gem lettuces
- 4 burger buns
- 2 shallots
- 2 free-range egg yolks
- 1 lemon

Directions

1. Heat 2 tablespoons of olive oil over a medium-low heat.
2. Add the shallots, garlic, and chili let cook until softened.
3. Blend the cod, scoop into a bowl, with crabmeat, stir to combine.

4. Add the prawns to the bowl of shallot mixture. Season.
5. Mold the mixture into patties.
6. Refrigerate for 45 minutes.
7. Whisk the egg yolks and lemon juice into a bowl with sunflower oil.
8. Stir in the wasabi until combined, season with a pinch of sea salt. Stir in the rocket, refrigerate.
9. Thread the lettuces onto a large barbecue skewer.
10. Brush the seafood patties with a little oil and barbecue for 3 minutes.
11. Toast the burger buns briefly.
12. Serve and enjoy.

Japanese inspired Mediterranean Seafood salad

Ingredients

- 1 squid, cleaned
- Olive oil
- ½ tablespoon of soy sauce
- 250g of cooked octopus
- 8 large cooked peeled prawns
- 1 handful of salad leaves
- 1 small handful of edible flowers
- 1 tablespoon of sesame seeds
- 3 tablespoons of toasted sesame oil
- 1 tablespoon yuzu juice
- 1 teaspoon of togarashi spice mix

Directions

1. Heat ½ tablespoon of olive oil over a medium heat.
2. Cook the squid for 4 minutes.
3. Add soy sauce over high heat, stir continuously for 2 minutes.
4. Transfer to a salad bowl.

5. Toast the sesame seeds in a dry frying pan until golden, combine with sesame seeds, sesame oil, yuzu juice, and togarashi spice mix.
6. Place sliced octopus with prawns in the salad bowl.
7. Serve and enjoy with edible flowers.

Prawn and chorizo orzo

Ingredients

- 400ml of passata
- 400g of large cooked peeled king prawns
- 200g of quality chorizo
- 200g of cherry tomatoes
- 300g of orzo
- ½ a bunch of fresh basil
- 4 tablespoons of olive oil
- 2 cloves of garlic
- 2 tablespoons of sherry vinegar

Directions

1. Preheat the oven to 350°F.
2. Heat half of olive oil, fry the garlic with chorizo for 3 minutes.
3. Deglaze the pan with the vinegar.
4. Add the passata with orzo and water boil, lower heat let simmer 15 minutes, stirring occasionally.
5. Spread the cherry tomatoes over a baking tray, drizzled with the rest of the olive oil, season.
6. Roast for until soft.
7. Stir half the basil into the pasta, along with the prawns.

8. Serve and enjoy.

Prawns with fennel

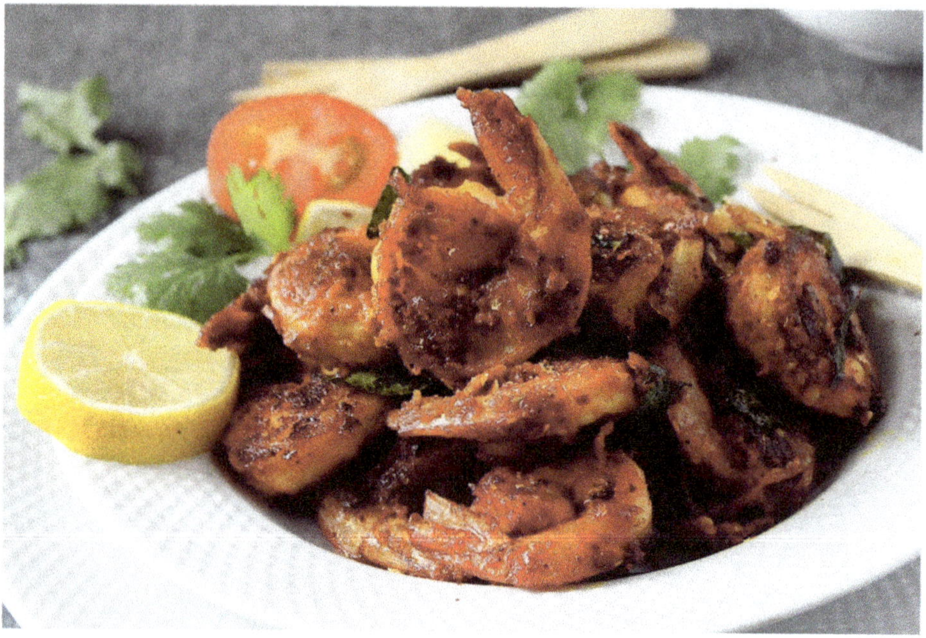

Ingredients

- 10 large raw prawns
- Sprigs of fresh flat-leaf parsley
- Olive oil
- 750g of ripe cherry tomatoes
- 1 lemon
- 1 bulb of fennel
- 1 large wineglass of white wine
- 2 cloves of garlic

Directions

1. Heat olive oil and fry the garlic till golden.
2. Add the fennel and parsley stalks, sauté for 10 minutes over low heat.
3. Add tomatoes to the pan with the wine, let boil and simmer for 10 minutes.
4. Add prawns to the pan, let cook for 4 minutes or until cooked and pink.
5. Stir through parsley leaves and season.
6. Serve and enjoy with lemon wedges.

Love dumplings

Ingredients

- Sprigs of fresh basil
- Sprigs of fresh mint
- 1 lime
- 1 large shallot
- 4 tablespoons of fish sauce
- 2 cloves of garlic
- 4 spring onions
- ½ a bunch of fresh coriander
- 200g of raw peeled prawns
- 4 tablespoons of caster sugar
- 16 round dumpling wrappers
- 1 fresh red chili
- 100g of glass noodles
- Chili sauce
- 1 tablespoon of unsalted peanuts
- 1 lettuce

Directions

1. Combine chili, lime juice, sugar, fish sauce, and water.
2. Dunk in a cute bowl, save the rest for dressing lettuce, herb and noodle salad.

3. Place the prawns together with the shallot, garlic, coriander, and the whites of the spring onions in a bowl.
4. Season with black pepper and a pinch of sea salt, mix.
5. Lay out your wrappers and spoon a teaspoon of filling into the middle of each.
6. Brush the edges of one wrapper with water, fold in half, then pleat and pinch the edges together to secure. Repeat for the rest.
7. Place an oiled pan over a medium heat.
8. Add the dumplings with a splash of water, and cover for 3 minutes.
9. Cook noodles according to the packet Directions.
10. Toast, and crush the peanuts.
11. Serve and enjoy.

Mushroom cannelloni

Ingredients

- 250g of dried cannelloni tubes
- 120g of Cheddar cheese
- 2 cloves of garlic
- 2 leeks
- 1-liter semi-skimmed milk
- 2 small onions
- 750g of shell nut mushrooms
- 75g of plain flour
- Olive oil

Directions

1. Preheat your oven ready to 350°F.
2. Pulse the onions with garlic in a food processor.
3. Add into a large casserole pan on a medium-high heat with olive oil.
4. Add pulsed leeks with mushroom, stir into the pan.
5. Let cook for 15 minutes, stirring regularly.
6. Season to perfection.
7. Pour 3 tablespoons of olive oil into another different pan over a medium heat.

8. Whisk in the flour and milk, let simmer for 5 minutes, add cheese and season.
9. Pour 1/3 of the sauce into roasting tray.
10. Push both ends of each pasta tube into it to fill, lining them up in the tray.
11. Pour over the rest of the sauce, slice the reserved mushrooms for decoration.
12. Drizzle with olive oil.
13. Let bake for 45 minutes.
14. Serve and enjoy.

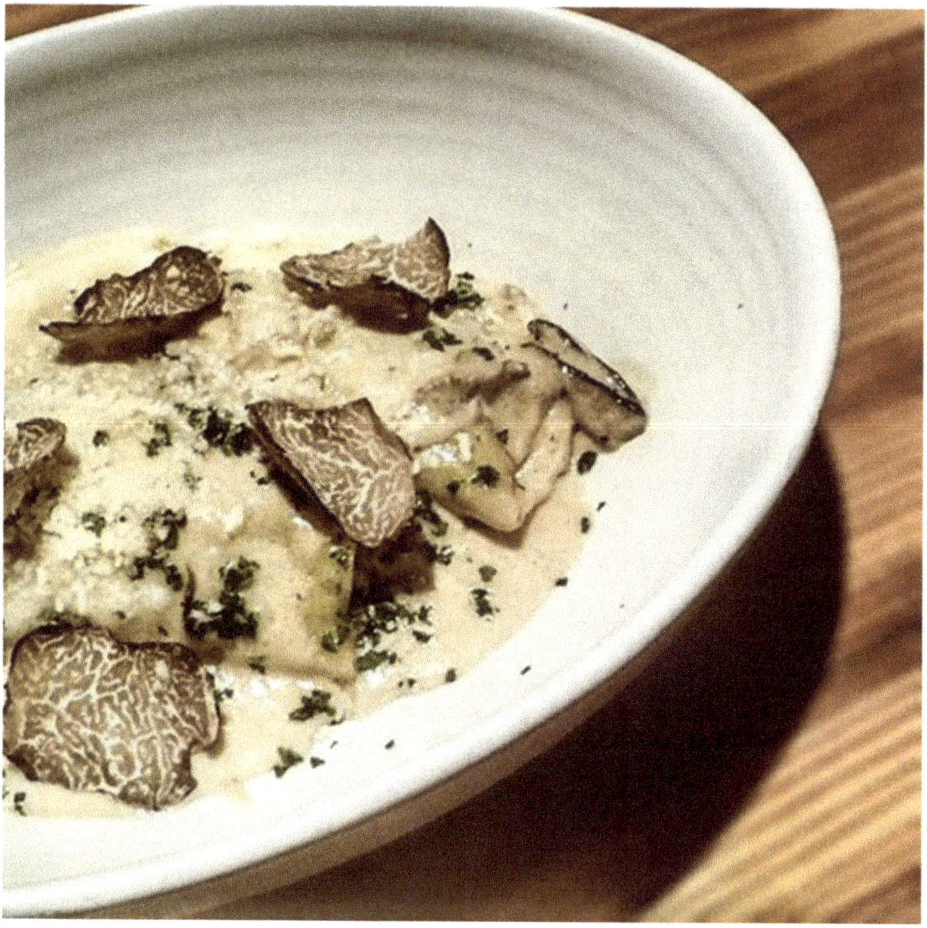

Mushroom stroganoff

Ingredients

- 1 tablespoon of baby capers
- 50ml of whisky
- 1 red onion
- 2 cloves of garlic
- 80g of half-fat crème fraiche
- Smoked paprika
- 4 silver skin pickled onions
- 2 cornichons
- 400g of mixed mushrooms
- 4 sprigs of fresh flat-leaf parsley
- Olive oil

Directions

1. Place a large non-stick frying pan over a high heat.
2. Place in the mushrooms together with the red onions, shake into one layer, dry-fry for 5 minutes, stirring regularly.
3. Drizzle in olive oil.
4. Add the garlic together with the pickled onions, parsley stalks, cornichons, and capers.
5. Shortly, pour in the whisky, tilt the pan to flame,

6. Then, add ¼ of a teaspoon of paprika together with the crème fraiche and parsley, toss.
7. Season with sea salt and black pepper.
8. Divide between plates, sprinkle over a little paprika.
9. Serve and enjoy with fluffy rice.

Mushroom toad in the hole

Ingredients

- Red wine vinegar
- 4 free-range large eggs
- 4 sprigs of rosemary
- 175g of plain flour
- 2 cloves of garlic
- 175ml of whole milk
- 4 large Portobello mushrooms
- 2 onions
- 250ml of smooth porter
- Olive oil

Directions

1. Preheat your oven to 400°F.
2. Whisk the eggs with flour, a pinch of sea salt, milk, and bit of water into a smooth batter.
3. Place the mushrooms cap side down in a large non-stick roasting tray.
4. Drizzle with olive oil.
5. Season with salt and black pepper.
6. Let roast for 30 minutes.

7. Place onions and sliced mushroom peelings, some rosemary in a pan on a medium-low heat with bit of olive oil.
8. Let cook for 15 minutes, stirring occasionally.
9. Add the porter with red wine vinegar, stir in the remaining flour shortly.
10. Season, add garlic, remaining rosemary, drizzle, rub with a little olive oil.
11. Remove the tray, pour the batter into the tray, place mushrooms close to the center.
12. Sprinkle over the oiled garlic and rosemary.
13. Place in oven for 25 minutes.
14. Serve and enjoy with gravy.

Wild mushroom and venison stroganoff

Ingredients

- 1 knob of butter
- 1 onion
- 1 clove of garlic
- Extra virgin olive oil
- 150ml of soured cream
- 250g of mixed wild mushrooms
- 1 lemon
- 1 teaspoon of sweet paprika
- 150g of basmati rice
- ½ a bunch of fresh flat-leaf parsley
- 1 handful of cornichons
- 300g of venison saddle
- Gin

Directions

1. Cook the rice per the package Directions, until just undercooked.
2. Drain any excess water. Steam covered till ready.

3. Place the onion and garlic with olive oil into a large frying pan over a medium heat, cook for 5 minutes.
4. Stir the paprika into the pan with the mushrooms, let cook for 5 minutes.
5. Season the venison with sea salt and black pepper.
6. Fry meat for 1 minute.
7. Add and flame the gin, stir in the butter with gratings of lemon zest and lemon juice.
8. Stir in most of the soured cream, season, let simmer for 1 minute.
9. Swirl through the remaining soured cream, scatter over the sliced cornichons and parsley.
10. Sprinkle with a pinch of paprika.
11. Serve and enjoy immediately.

Crispy mushroom shawarma

Ingredients

- 4 tablespoons of tahini
- 800g of Portobello and oyster mushrooms
- 1 red onion
- 2 tablespoons of dukkha
- 2 cloves of garlic
- 1 teaspoon of ground allspice
- Olive oil
- 2 tablespoons of pomegranate molasses
- 200g of natural yoghurt
- 10 radishes
- 1 teaspoon of ground cumin
- ½ cucumber
- 100g of ripe cherry tomatoes
- 1 tablespoon white wine vinegar
- 2 preserved lemons
- 1 teaspoon of smoked paprika
- 200g jar of pickled jalapeño chilies
- 1 bunch of fresh mint
- 4 large flatbreads

Directions

1. Sieve yogurt into a bowl.
2. Place Portobello mushrooms, onion, garlic, and lemons, and bash in a mortar with olive oil, black pepper, and allspices.
3. Muddle and toss with all the mushrooms and onions, let marinate overnight.
4. Preheat the oven to /475°F.
5. Place mushrooms and onions on a large baking tray, roast for 20 minutes, turning occasionally.
6. Drizzle over the pomegranate molasses for the last 3 minutes.
7. Toss the cucumber, radishes, and tomatoes with a pinch of salt and the vinegar.
8. Combine jalapeños and mint leaves, bend until fine.
9. Pour back into the jar
10. Warm the flatbreads, spread with tahini, sprinkle with pickled vegetables, remaining mint leaves and dukkha.
11. Carve and scatter over the gnarly vegetables, dollop over yoghurt.
12. Roll up, slice and enjoy.

Pithivier pie

Ingredients

- Olive oil
- 800ml of semi-skimmed milk
- 2 x 320g sheets of all-butter puff pastry
- 1 large free-range egg
- 2 large leeks
- 1 knob of unsalted butter
- 2 cloves of garlic
- 1 bunch of fresh flat-leaf parsley
- 400g of mixed mushrooms
- 75g of plain flour
- 120g of blue cheese
- 2 teaspoons of English mustard
- 1 whole celeriac

Directions

1. Preheat the oven to 400°F.
2. Roast the celeriac for 1 hour and 30 minutes.
3. Slice and season with sea salt and black pepper.
4. Place leeks, mushroom, garlic, and butter in a large casserole pan on a medium heat, cook for 15 minutes.

5. Stir in the flour, mustard, milk, let simmer for 5 minutes, stirring regularly.
6. Stir in the parsley, crumble in the cheese, season when off heat.
7. Line bowl with Clingfilm.
8. Arrange slices of celeriac in and around the bowl until covered, layer with the remaining celeriac in the bowl, finishing with celeriac.
9. Pull over the Clingfilm, weigh it down, refrigerate overnight with the remaining sauce.
10. Preheat the oven to 350°F.
11. On greaseproof paper, roll both sheets of pastry out to around.
12. Unwrap the filling parcel and place in the middle of one sheet.
13. Beat the egg and brush around the edge of the pastry and celeriac.
14. Lay the second piece of pastry on top, smoothing around the shape of the filling, seal.
15. Bake at the bottom of the oven for 2 hours.
16. Serve an enjoy.

Midnight pan-cooked breakfast

Ingredients

- Crusty bread
- Sausages
- Mushrooms
- Olive oil
- Higher-welfare smoked
- Ripe tomatoes
- Large free-range eggs

Directions

1. Preheat your pan to high heat.
2. Place sausages in the pan at one side.
3. Place a pile of mushrooms over the pan with olive oil.
4. Coat the mushrooms with oil, season with sea salt and black pepper.
5. Push to one side, then lay some slices of bacon and halved tomatoes in the pan.
6. Cook for briefly until the bacon is crisp, flip the bacon over.
7. Add 3 eggs at different ends of the pan dribbling around the sausages, bacon, tomatoes and mushrooms.
8. Lower the heat, continue to cook for 1 minute.
9. Serve and enjoy.

Garlic mushroom pasta

Ingredients

- 2 cloves of garlic
- 2 heaped tablespoons of half-fat crème fraiche
- 250g of mixed mushrooms
- 150g of dried toffee
- 25g of Parmesan cheese

Directions

1. Cook the pasta in a pan of boiling salted water per the package Directions.
2. Drain and reserve some cooking water for later.
3. Place garlic, olive oil, mushrooms in a large non-stick frying pan on a medium.
4. Season with sea salt and black pepper, let cook for 8 minutes, tossing regularly.
5. Toss the drained pasta into the mushroom pan with a splash of reserved cooking water.
6. Add grated Parmesan with crème fraiche.
7. Taste, and adjust the seasoning.
8. Serve and enjoy.

Baked garlicky mushrooms

Ingredients

- 40g of Cheddar cheese
- 4 cloves of garlic
- 350g of ripped mixed-color cherry tomatoes
- 4 large Portobello mushrooms
- ½ a bunch of fresh sage

Directions

1. Preheat the oven to 400°F.
2. Place mushrooms in a roasting tray, drizzle with olive oil and red wine vinegar.
3. Add a pinch of sea salt and black pepper and toss.
4. Place in garlic and sage leaves, sit the mushrooms stalk side up on the top.
5. Let bake for 10 minutes.
6. Remove the tray, crumble the cheese into the mushroom cups and sprinkle over the reserved garlic and sage.
7. Return to the oven for 15 more minutes.
8. Serve and enjoy.

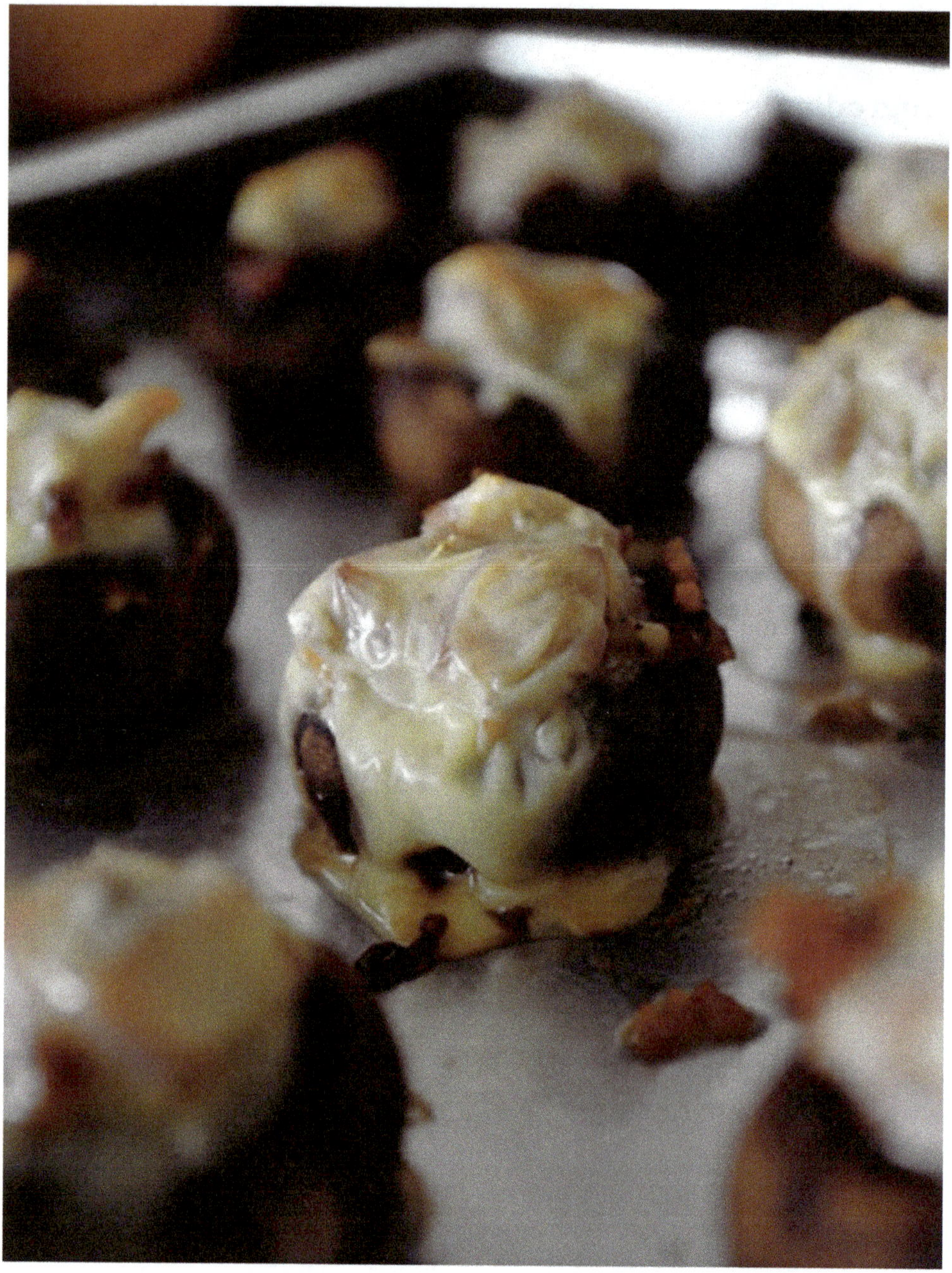

CPSIA information can be obtained
at www.ICGtesting.com
Printed in the USA
LVHW051654010621
689062LV00009B/563